Prostate Cancer Cookbook For Seniors

A Recipe Book For A Healthy And Happy Life

By

Dr. Anna R. Brown

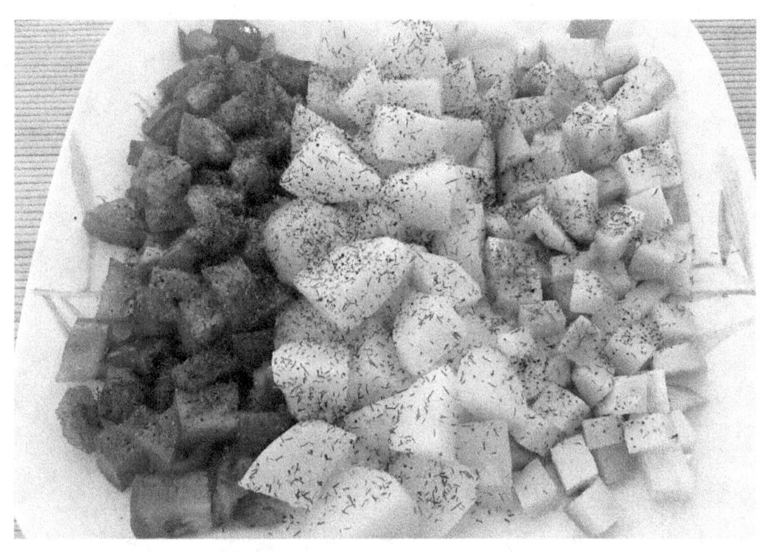

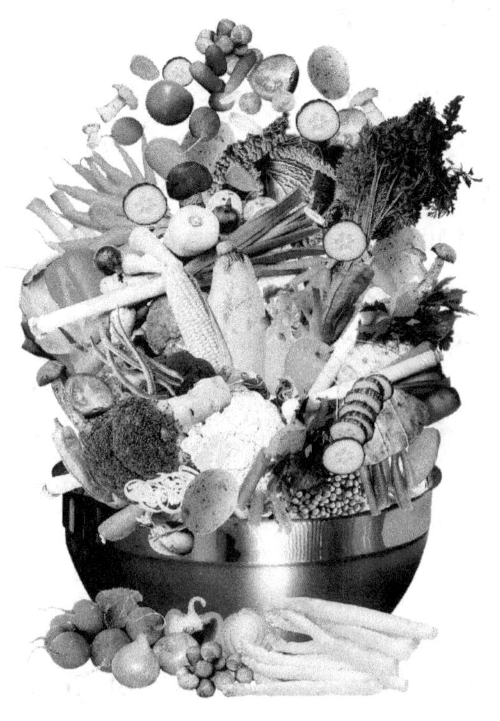

INTRODUCTION

Life was about to change dramatically for a community of retirees who had previously lived in a peaceful town surrounded by rolling hills. These people, coming from all walks of life, were about to confront a terrible foe: prostate cancer. The disease shook him to his very core, destroying the serenity and relaxation he had come to value in his accustomed routine. Their futures were uncertain as they sought solace and guidance.

Despite the enormous enormity of the crisis, these courageous retirees did not give up hope. They set out on their journey with bravery and determination, confident in their ability to shape their future. They needed information, a support group, and the freedom to make choices that would better their health. During this period of profound change, the concept of a cookbook tailored for older adults diagnosed with prostate cancer emerged.

This cookbook is much more
than just a collection of recipes. It's a tribute to
the grit of the old. In addition to satisfying your
curiosity, it may also serve as a roadmap to
expanding your horizons. Each paragraph is a
guiding beacon that illuminates the path to
happiness.

In this cookbook, you'll discover a ton of recipes
that support prostate cancer and older people's
well-being. These recipes were carefully created,
taking into account the special nutritional needs
and challenges experienced by those with
prostate cancer. By fusing flavor and nutrition
into a seamless symphony, they celebrate food as
medicine.

This cookbook is not only a collection of
delicious recipes, however. It is evidence of the
strength of collaboration and common interests.
You will hear tales from seniors who have gone
before you as you embark on this trip. They will
motivate you and serve as a reminder that you
are not fighting this battle alone. Your resolve to
directly combat prostate cancer will be

strengthened by their stories of tenacity and accomplishment.

Flipping through the pages will take you to cozy kitchens full of affection. You'll see the joy of elders getting together, telling tales, and exchanging skills and advice. Since they have been handed down through the generations, these recipes have preserved ancient knowledge while incorporating modern nutritional understanding.

These recipes include the key to healthy eating and recovery. Each component has been carefully chosen based on its ability to improve prostate health. Each meal is intended to create a symphony of tastes that will delight your taste buds and energize your body. Each recipe has been carefully prepared to provide a symphony of tastes, from the vivid hues of antioxidant-rich fruits and vegetables to the robust richness of lean meats and entire grains.

However, there is more than just physical nutrition included in this cookbook. The nourishment of the soul is another issue. It gives you the motivation to embrace life's basic pleasures, discover joy wherever you are, and take pleasure in making and sharing meals with those you care about. It serves as a reminder that food can maintain both your physical and mental health.

Dear Readers, be aware that you are not traveling alone as you start this culinary journey. The Prostate Cancer Cookbook for Seniors is a monument to our collective fortitude and fortitude. The route to a better, full life is illuminated by prostate cancer, despite the obstacles it presents.

In these pages, you'll find tales, recipes, and a sense of community that may help you grow. This cookbook should go with you on your journey, giving you nourishment, encouragement, and the unwavering conviction that you have what it takes to triumph against prostate cancer with dignity and tenacity.

This recipe should be a reminder of the resilient nature of older adults worldwide.

Chapter 1

A Diagnosis That Changes Lives

Now and again, life gives us a curveball that tosses all we know to the wind. A prostate cancer diagnosis is one such surprise, and it may be especially painful for seniors. Prostate cancer is a common illness that affects millions of men worldwide. There is, however, hope, and this cookbook attempts to serve as a guide for elders dealing with the problems of prostate cancer. Let me tell you a tale of Henry, a man who was diagnosed with Prostate Cancer.

A guy called Henry formerly lived in a beautiful neighborhood filled with bright gardens and friendly neighbors. Henry was a senior citizen who was quietly enjoying the pace of his retirement. He loved caring for his garden, going on walks in the park, and spending time with his family.

But Henry's life was flipped upside down one tragic day. He was given a diagnosis that would change the direction of his life forever: prostate cancer. This revelation sent a flood of emotions crashing down on him, like a sudden storm on a clear day—shock, dread, and a deep feeling of uncertainty.

As Henry sat in the doctor's office, listening to the words that reverberated around the room, a rush of questions washed over him. What caused this to happen? What does this indicate for his prospects? Most importantly, what actions might he take to combat this sickness and reclaim control of his health?

Henry went through the crowded streets after leaving the doctor's office, his mind absorbed by his diagnosis. He realized he couldn't undertake this voyage alone; he needed direction, support, and a ray of hope to help him traverse the uncharted region ahead. During this soul-searching trek, he came across a little bookshop.

Henry was drawn inside by an unseen force, met by the aroma of newly printed pages and the whispered murmurs of many tales waiting to be revealed. As he browsed the shelves, his gaze was drawn to a book titled "Prostate Cancer Cookbook for Seniors." He stretched out, intrigued, and gingerly grasped the book in his hand as if it contained the answers he needed.

When Henry opened the book, he was plunged into a universe of knowledge and opportunity. The pages were packed with stories of seniors who had overcome similar challenges. They spoke about resilience, optimism, and the transforming effect of feeding one's body via the art of cooking.

Henry started to read, enthralled by tales that spoke to him about his own life. He discovered that prostate cancer was a path shared by many, with each person confronting unique problems but linked by a similar goal—reclaiming their health and finding pleasure every day.

Henry uncovered a treasure mine of information regarding prostate cancer—the origins, symptoms, and treatment options—within the pages. He discovered how nutrition and lifestyle modifications may help him on his path and perhaps enhance his results. But it was the painstakingly produced dishes that comprised the heart and soul of the cookbook that sparked a flame of optimism inside him.

Each meal was meticulously developed to nurture his body and spirit, from colorful breakfast bowls brimming with antioxidants to soothing soups and stews filled with nutrients. The cookbook recognized the power of whole foods, relying on the knowledge of previous generations to create meals that were both tasty and fulfilling.

Henry saw himself in his kitchen, surrounded by the calming fragrances of herbs and spices, preparing a prostate cancer-friendly dinner for himself and his loved ones. He observed his family gathered around the table, exchanging tales and laughing, finding peace in the simple act of sharing food.

Henry realized, armed with increased information and energy, that his diagnosis, although frightening, was not the end of his tale. He saw that his prostate cancer path could be one of resistance, progress, and success. He had a newfound sense of purpose and drive to confront the difficulties ahead after reading the Prostate Cancer Cookbook for Seniors.

A wave of appreciation flooded over Henry as he closed the book. Gratitude to the writers who put their hearts and souls into establishing a resource that will alter the lives of seniors suffering from g prostate cancer for the rest of their lives. Gratitude for his loved ones' constant support

Section 1: Understanding Prostate Cancer

Chapter 2

The Prostate and Its Role in Men's Health.

The prostate gland, located deep inside a man's body, is a fascinating organ that is crucial to men's health. This walnut-shaped gland may be little, but it has a huge impact on a man's health and happiness.

The urethra, through which urine and sperm travel, is placed slightly below the bladder, and the prostate gland surrounds it. Its main job is to secrete seminal fluid, which helps sperm survive and travel throughout the ejaculatory process. The prostate produces a fluid that improves the viability of sperm and makes fertilization more likely.

The prostate gland is important to men's urinary health for reasons beyond reproduction. Because of its proximity to the urethra, the prostate may disrupt regular urination if it undergoes any kind of aberrant alteration. An enlarged prostate, for example, might put pressure on the urethra, causing urinary issues including the need to urinate often, poor urine flow, or the sensation that one's bladder isn't empty.

As men age, prostate health becomes more important to them, mostly because of the risk of prostate cancer. It's important to remember, nevertheless, that not all prostate anomalies indicate malignancy. Benign prostatic hyperplasia (BPH), sometimes known as an enlarged prostate but not malignant, is a common prostate disorder. It is important to be checked out if you have any symptoms related to your urinary system, since BPH may create symptoms that are similar to those of prostate cancer.

Because of its prevalence in males, early identification of prostate cancer is essential for successful treatment. Digital rectal exams (DRE) and blood tests for prostate-specific antigen (PSA) should be performed routinely to assist identify anomalies that may need further study. Just because you were diagnosed with prostate cancer doesn't mean your life has to stop being rewarding. Many men with prostate cancer now have a decent quality of life because of advances in medical science and a holistic approach to treatment.

Prostatitis, inflammation of the prostate gland, may develop in addition to cancer and BPH. Symptoms of this disorder include bladder issues, pain, and discomfort, and may be brought on by infection or other circumstances. Prostatitis requires immediate medical treatment to treat and relieve its symptoms.

The ability to take charge of one's health is greatly enhanced by knowledge about the prostate gland and its complex function in male health. Although it may be impossible to prevent all prostate issues, some measures may be taken to improve prostate health and lessen the likelihood of complications.

It's crucial to stick to a healthy routine. Maintaining a healthy weight, eating a diet full of fruits and vegetables, whole grains, lean proteins, and healthy fats, and engaging in regular physical activity may all help men preserve prostate health. These habits are good for the prostate, but they also promote overall health and help ward off other chronic conditions.

Urologists and other medical specialists should be consulted often to keep an eye on prostate health and catch any problems in their earliest stages. Urinary symptoms, changes in sexual function, or other issues connected to the prostate should be discussed openly with healthcare practitioners to ensure prompt diagnosis and treatment.

As we continue our journey through this cookbook, we will learn how proper diet may improve general health and prostate function. Taking care of our bodies and ensuring the prostate gland continues to function normally may be accomplished via a combination of prostate cancer-friendly meals and a health-conscious approach to meal planning.

Let's go on an adventure of self-improvement and healthy eating as we learn to harness the power of a diet that's good for your prostate. We can take responsibility for our health, embrace a life of energy and longevity, and appreciate the importance of the prostate in men's health by learning about its function and making informed decisions.

Chapter 3

Prostate Cancer: Causes, Symptoms, and Treatment Options

Prostate cancer is a strong foe in the delicate web of men's health. Numerous lives might be adversely affected by this pernicious illness, which can silently establish itself within the prostate gland. The fight against prostate cancer requires understanding the causes, identifying the symptoms, and researching the many treatment choices.

Causes of Prostate Cancer.

Although the precise causes of prostate cancer are still unknown, certain risk factors have been discovered. The risk of prostate cancer significantly rises beyond the age of 50, making aging a key determinant. A person's chance of developing prostate cancer is increased by a family history, thus genetic factors are also important. Men of African origin have a greater incidence of prostate cancer, and ethnicity also increases risk.

It's important to recognize that although these variables may make prostate cancer more likely, they do not ensure its development. While many people without these risk factors are given a prostate cancer diagnosis, other people with several risk factors never get the condition. This demonstrates the intricate interaction between genetics, the environment, and lifestyle decisions that cause prostate cancer.

Symptoms of Prostate Cancer

In its early stages, prostate cancer seldom shows any outward signs. It may be difficult to identify because of this, which highlights the need for routine screening. However, as the condition advances, a variety of symptoms may become apparent, such as:

Alterations to Urinary Function: Urinating often, particularly during sleep (nocturia), having a weak urine flow, having trouble initiating or terminating urination, and feeling that one's bladder isn't completely emptied.

Bleeding Disorders The appearance of blood in the urine (hematuria) or semen (hematospermia) may be a marker of prostate cancer, while it may also be caused by other illnesses.

Erectile Dysfunction: Prostate cancer may affect sexual function, making it hard to get or keep an erection.

Discomfort may occur in several parts of the body if prostate cancer has progressed to an advanced stage. This discomfort might be constant or it can come and go.

Bear in mind that these signs and symptoms are not exclusive to prostate cancer and may be brought on by a variety of other health issues. However, it is critical to see a doctor for a thorough assessment and diagnosis if any of these symptoms continue or create worry.

Treatment Options for Prostate Cancer:

The stage and severity of the disease, the individual's general health and age, and personal preferences all influence prostate cancer therapy. Among the treatment options available are:

Active Surveillance: Active surveillance may be suggested for early-stage, slow-growing prostate cancer. Regular monitoring using PSA testing, digital rectal exams (DRE), and biopsies aid in tracking the evolution of the illness and determining the need for intervention.

Surgery: To eradicate malignant cells, the prostate gland may be surgically removed (prostatectomy). Different surgical procedures, such as open surgery or minimally invasive techniques like laparoscopic or robotic-assisted surgery, may be used depending on the degree and severity of the malignancy.

Radiation Therapy: High-energy radiation is used to target and kill cancer cells in this therapy. It may be delivered externally (external beam radiation treatment) or internally (brachytherapy) by inserting radioactive sources directly into the prostate.

Hormone Therapy: Male hormones, notably testosterone, are required for the proliferation of prostate cancer cells. Hormone treatment tries to reduce or prevent cancer development by suppressing the production or effect of certain hormones. This may be accomplished with drugs or by surgically removing the testicles (orchiectomy).

Chemotherapy may be indicated if the cancer has progressed beyond the prostate gland or if previous therapies have been unsuccessful. Chemotherapy is a treatment that employs strong medications to target and eliminate cancer cells throughout the body.

Immunotherapy: This novel therapeutic method uses the body's immune system to locate and destroy cancer cells. Immunotherapy may boost the immune system's capacity to recognize and kill prostate cancer cells.
It's important to remember that each person's circumstance is unique, and treatment approaches should be customized to their exact

requirements. Healthcare providers, such as urologists and oncologists, play an important role in assisting patients through the decision-making process and proposing the best treatment choices depending on the stage and features of the cancer.

Furthermore, complementary and supportive therapies such as dietary counseling, pain management, and psychological support may improve general well-being and increase the efficacy of traditional treatments.

A prostate cancer diagnosis may be frightening, but because of advances in medical research and a multidisciplinary approach to therapy, the future for many people is bright. Maintaining open lines of contact with healthcare practitioners, asking questions, and seeking help from loved ones and support groups are critical.

As we continue through this cookbook, we will look at how diet may help promote prostate health and improve treatment results. We may fuel our bodies, enhance general well-being, and add gastronomic joy to the treatment path by adopting a prostate cancer-friendly diet and implementing the delectable dishes on these pages.

Let us walk this journey together, arming ourselves with information and embracing the opportunities that await us. We can tackle prostate cancer with fortitude, optimism, and a willingness to live our lives to the fullest if we understand the reasons, recognize the symptoms, and investigate the available treatment choices.

Section 2: The Role of Diet in Prostate Cancer

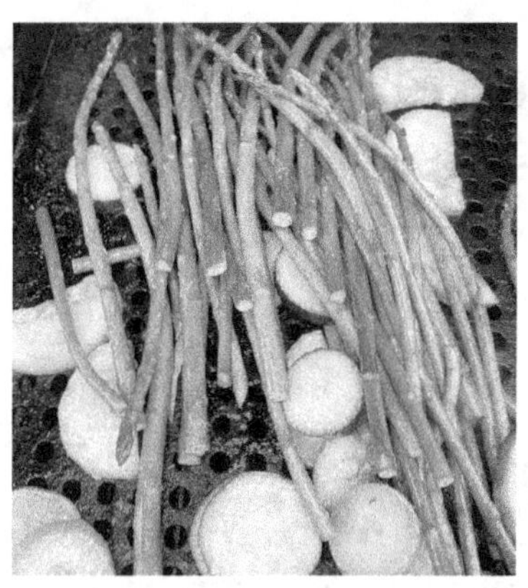

Chapter 4: The Impact of Diet on Prostate Cancer.

The importance of a balanced diet in the pursuit of health and happiness is hard to overestimate. The diets of those coping with prostate cancer are no different from those of anybody else, in that the food we eat plays an essential part in maintaining the body's activities. The more we learn about the link between food and prostate cancer, the more equipped we will be to use nutrition as a weapon in the battle against the illness.

Prostate cancer cannot be prevented or cured by changing one's diet, but studies have shown that certain dietary patterns and certain nutrients may affect one's chance of acquiring prostate cancer, the course of the illness, and the success of therapy. The likelihood of problems, the efficacy of therapies, and the body's ability to recover are all improved by eating a prostate cancer-friendly diet.

So, what exactly does a diet that helps those with prostate cancer consist of? Let's break it down and see how it relates to your diet.

Accept plant-based foods: Several research has shown that a diet high in plant-based foods has anti-prostate cancer-preventive effects. A variety of vitamins, minerals, antioxidants, phytochemicals, and other nutrients found in fruits, vegetables, legumes, whole grains, and nuts have anti-inflammatory and anticancer qualities. Aim to pile as many different leafy greens, cruciferous veggies (including broccoli, cauliflower, and Brussels sprouts), berries, tomatoes, and citrus fruits as you can onto your plate.

Make Healthy Fats Your Top Priority: Choose healthy fats that promote general health and minimize inflammation. Fatty fish (salmon, mackerel, and sardines), flaxseeds, chia seeds, and walnuts are examples of sources of omega-3 fatty acids. Include monounsaturated fats, which are included in foods like avocados, olive oil, and almonds. In addition to supporting cardiovascular health, these fats may also be protective against prostate cancer.

Cut down on your intake of red and processed meats, since there seems to be a correlation between these foods and an increased risk of prostate cancer. Dietary red meats and processed meats like bacon, sausage, and deli meats should be consumed in moderation. Select skinless fowl and fish as well as lentils and tofu as healthy plant-based protein choices.

Select Whole Grains Instead of Refined Flour Whole grains are the healthiest option since they include the highest levels of beneficial nutrients, fiber, and phytochemicals. Brown rice, quinoa, whole wheat, oats, and barley are all examples of whole grains that provide a steady stream of energy and are good for your digestive system. They are an important part of a healthy diet because they help you feel full for longer.

Maintaining a healthy fluid balance is crucial to your body functioning properly. Water helps your cells work, your digestive system runs smoothly, and your body gets rid of waste products, therefore it's important to drink enough of it throughout the day. Reduce your intake of sugary drinks like soda, energy drinks, and juices with added sugar if you're trying to lose weight.

Moderate Alcohol drinking: Although there may be some health advantages to moderate alcohol use, excessive alcohol drinking has been related to an increased risk of prostate cancer. If you decide to consume alcohol, do it sensibly and by advice. Men who drink moderately generally consume up to two alcoholic drinks daily.

Prostate cancer-fighting nutrients should be consumed:
In promoting prostate health and preventing prostate cancer, several foods have shown promise. Lycopene (found in tomatoes and watermelon), selenium (found in fish, whole grains, and Brazil nuts), vitamin E (found in foods like almonds, spinach, and sunflower seeds), and cruciferous veggies (like broccoli, cauliflower, and kale) that include substances like sulforaphane are a few of these. While these nutrients need to be a component of a balanced diet, it's crucial to keep in mind that they shouldn't be used in place of medical care and should only be taken as part of a comprehensive strategy for managing prostate cancer.

Seek Professional Advice: To obtain individualized dietary advice catered to your unique requirements and treatment plan, speak with a certified dietitian or nutritionist with expertise in oncology. They may provide helpful advice, assist you in overcoming dietary obstacles, and make sure that your dietary decisions are in line with your long-term health objectives.

It's crucial to remember that although food may help manage prostate cancer, it should be a part of an all-encompassing treatment strategy. Always heed the advice given to you by your medical team, which may include oncologists, urologists, and nutritionists.

We may feed our bodies and build a good attitude and proactive approach to our health by adopting a prostate cancer-friendly diet. Every meal offers the chance to make decisions that promote our health and strengthen our resistance to prostate cancer.

This cookbook's culinary trip will take us through a wide variety of mouthwatering dishes that have been carefully created to adhere to dietary guidelines that are conducive to preventing prostate cancer. Let's embrace the nutritious potential of each mouthful, harness the power of nutrition, and enjoy the flavors. One dish at a time, we may develop a proactive and health-conscious strategy for dealing with our prostate cancer.

Chapter 5: Superfoods for Prostate Health

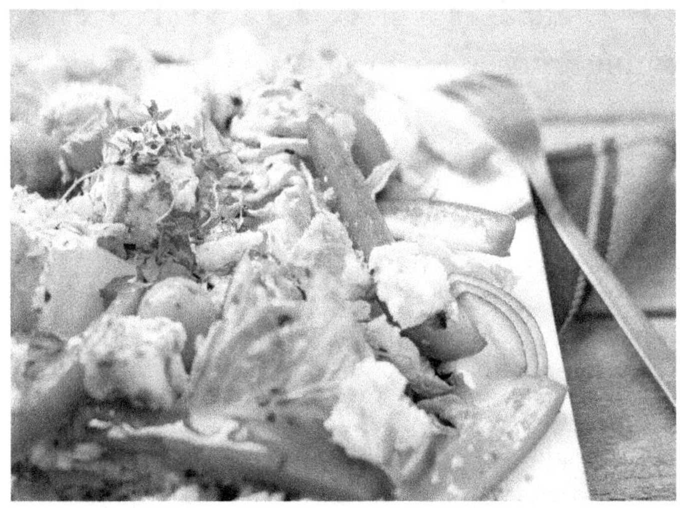

Due to their remarkable nutritional profiles and conceivable health advantages, several foods have come to be known as "superfoods" in the world of nutrition. By including these superfoods in your diet, you may give your body a beneficial boost of nutrients and other substances that could improve prostate health. Let's look at a few of these superfoods and how they could affect prostate health.

Tomatoes
Because of their high lycopene concentration, tomatoes are a prostate health powerhouse. The powerful antioxidant lycopene is what gives tomatoes their vivid red color. Lycopene may help lower the risk of prostate cancer and halt the disease's development, according to studies. Consider adding tomato-based sauces, soups, and stews to your meals as cooking tomatoes improves the absorption of lycopene.

Cruciferous veggies: Cruciferous veggies including broccoli, cauliflower, Brussels sprouts, and kale are a good source of vitamins, fiber, and glucosinolates. Sulforaphane, a substance found in these veggies, can slow the development of cancer cells and lower the risk of prostate cancer. Whether they are sautéed, roasted, or steamed, try to include a variety of these veggies into your diet.

Berries: Berries are rich in antioxidants, vitamins, and fiber. Some examples are strawberries, blueberries, raspberries, and blackberries. They provide a variety of health advantages, including possible protection against prostate cancer. Berries may be eaten as a snack, used in salads and desserts, or blended into smoothies.

Green tea: Green tea has long been valued for its ability to improve health. It has potent antioxidants called catechins that have been linked to a decreased incidence of prostate cancer. To get the potential advantages of green tea, drink a cup of it every day. Try replacing your usual cup of coffee with it if you like a hot beverage.

Fatty Fish: Omega-3 fatty acids, which have anti-inflammatory qualities, are abundant in fatty fish like salmon, mackerel, and sardines. These fats may improve overall prostate health and may lower the chance of prostate cancer. Aim to consume fatty fish a couple of times each week. If you don't eat fish, think about taking omega-3 supplements made from algae or other plant sources.

Nuts and seeds are a great source of healthy fats, fiber, and antioxidants. Some examples of nuts and seeds include almonds, walnuts, flaxseeds, and chia seeds. They provide a wholesome and practical snack choice that may benefit prostate health. To add crunch and nutrition to your meals, salads, or yogurt, add a handful of nuts or a dash of seeds.

Pomegranate: The possible anti-cancer benefits of pomegranates, notably their impact on prostate cancer, have drawn attention. Antioxidant-rich pomegranate juice and seeds may help slow the spread of cancer cells. Pomegranate juice is delicious. You may also add the seeds to salads or yogurt.

Products made from soy: Foods made from soy, such as tofu, tempeh, and soy milk, include substances called isoflavones that have been investigated for their ability to prevent prostate cancer. These substances are phytoestrogens, which resemble estrogen just somewhat. An advantageous complement to a prostate-healthy diet might be soy-based products, which can be used in moderation.

Keep in mind that including these superfoods in your diet should be a part of a larger, well-balanced eating strategy. It's crucial to concentrate on overall dietary habits and make decisions that prioritize whole, unprocessed meals while excluding processed items.

Chapter 6

The Power of Antioxidants and Phytochemicals

In the realm of nutrition, phytochemicals, and antioxidants well-being is a powerful friend in fostering health and wellbeing. These bioactive substances, which are mostly present in plant-based defenses essential for enhancing our bodies' natural defenses, preventing oxidative stress, and lowering our chance of developing chronic illnesses like prostate cancer. Let's investigate the benefits of phytochemicals and antioxidants and how they might support prostate health.

Understanding Antioxidants: Free radicals are unstable chemicals created naturally in the body that may harm our cells. Antioxidants are compounds that assist prevent this damage. Prostate cancer, among other illnesses, may arise as a result of free radicals' ability to generate oxidative stress and neutralized cells. These dangerous free radicals are neutralized by antioxidants, which lessen or stop their destructive effects.

Vitamins A, C, and E, as well as minerals like selenium and zinc, are all potent antioxidants. They are plentiful in whole grains, fruits, vegetables, nuts, seeds, and several spices. Our natural defense systems and prostate health may be supported by including foods high in antioxidants in our diets.

Phytochemicals and Their Benefits: Also referred to as phytonutrients, phytochemicals are physiologically active substances that are present in plants. They are in charge of giving fruits, vegetables, herbs, and spices their eye-catching colors, distinct scents, and distinctive flavors. Numerous health advantages of phytochemicals, such as their anti-inflammatory and antioxidant capabilities, may promote general health and may lower the risk of chronic illnesses like prostate cancer.

The effects of various phytochemicals on the body vary, and study is still being done to determine any possible health advantages. The following important phytochemicals have shown potential for supporting prostate health:

Lycopene is a powerful antioxidant that is most often found in tomatoes as well as other red-colored fruits like watermelon and grapefruit. Lycopene has been linked to a lower chance of developing prostate cancer. When tomatoes are cooked or processed into other items, the lycopene they contain becomes more readily available for absorption by the body.

Sulforaphane: Found in large quantities in cruciferous vegetables including kale, broccoli, cauliflower, and Brussels sprouts, sulforaphane has powerful anti-inflammatory and anti-cancer qualities. It could aid in preventing the development of prostate cancer cells and enhancing overall prostate health.

The key ingredient in turmeric is curcumin, which has potent anti-inflammatory and antioxidant effects. It has shown promise for limiting prostate cancer cell proliferation and decreasing body inflammation. Additionally supporting prostate health may be adding turmeric to your diet or taking pills containing curcumin.

Apples, onions, berries, and leafy greens are just a few examples of fruits and vegetables that contain antioxidant and anti-inflammatory quercetin. Prostate cancer risk may be decreased and cellular damage may be prevented.
Resveratrol is an antioxidant that may be found in grapes, berries, and red wine. Resveratrol is present in these foods because of their color. It is possible that it helps prevent cancer and contributes to the health of the prostate.

Antioxidants and Phytochemicals: How to Work Them Into Your Diet:
To get the most out of the benefits that antioxidants and phytochemicals provide for the health of your prostate, you should make it a priority to include in your diet a broad range of

colorful fruits, vegetables, whole grains, nuts, seeds, herbs, and spices. It is important to have a plant-based diet that includes a variety of fruits and vegetables of various colors since each kind of fruit and vegetable has a unique combination of antioxidants and phytochemicals.

Take into consideration the following recommendations to get the most out of your consumption of these healthful compounds:

You should pile a colorful selection of fruits and vegetables onto the other side of your dish. Aim for consuming at least five servings of vegetables and fruits every day, including a variety of dark green leafy vegetables, cruciferous vegetables, berries, and tomatoes.

Make sure that your diet includes a wide assortment of nuts and seeds. Include a handful of flaxseeds, almonds, or walnuts in one of your meals, or eat them on their own as a snack.

Choose brown rice, quinoa, whole wheat, and oats instead of refined grains like white rice or rolled oats since these grains are higher in fiber and antioxidants.

Make use of various herbs and spices in your food preparation. Cinnamon, ginger, turmeric, and garlic are all excellent sources of antioxidants, and turmeric also has anti-inflammatory qualities.

Choose plant-based forms of protein such as legumes, tofu, tempeh, and edamame instead of animal-based sources of protein since they provide a wider variety of phytochemicals in addition to the nutrients that the body needs.

Benefit from the antioxidant properties of a range of teas, including green tea, herbal tea, and other types of tea.

To get the benefits of the anti-oxidant element resveratrol, include in your diet either a modest number of red grapes or a glass of red wine (if doing so is not detrimental to your health).

It is essential to keep in mind that, even though antioxidants and phytochemicals may be beneficial to one's health, it is ideal to include them in one's diet in the context of a well-rounded and diverse eating plan. Whole foods often provide greater health benefits than isolated supplements because of the way diverse nutrients and chemicals interact together to create a synergistic effect.

You can provide your body with a spectrum of antioxidants and phytochemicals that promote prostate health and general well-being if you eat a colorful and diversified array of plant-based meals. These nutrients can be found in a wide variety of plant-based foods. You may make use of these naturally occurring substances as friends in your battle against prostate cancer and your quest to achieve optimum health.

Section3:

Recipes for Nourishment and Delight

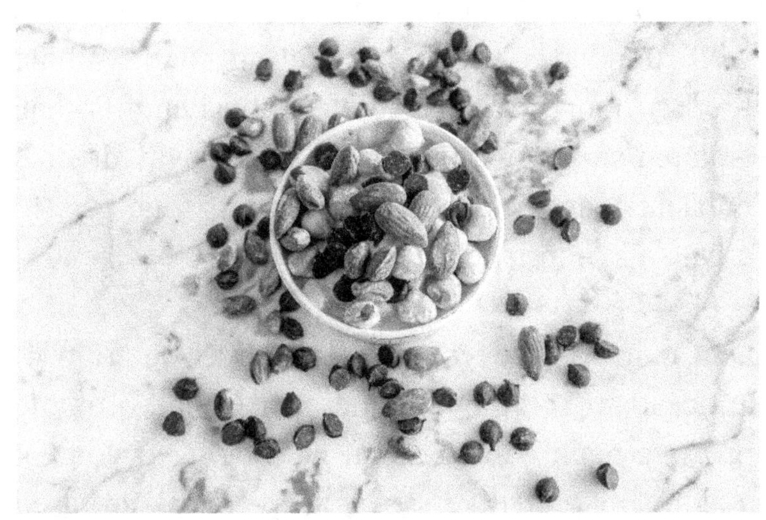

Chapter 6: Breakfast Recipes for a Healthy Start

Greek Yogurt Parfait With Granola

Spinach and Mushroom Frittata:Peanut Butter and Banana Smoothie:

Veggie Breakfast Scramble:

Avocado Toast with Poached Eggs:

A nourishing breakfast sets the tone for the day. In this chapter, we'll present a variety of prostate cancer-friendly breakfast recipes that are not only packed with essential nutrients but also delicious and satisfying. From hearty oatmeal bowls to energizing smoothies, seniors will find an array of options to kick-start their mornings.

Greek Yogurt Parfait With Granola

INGREDIENTS

1 cup plain Greek yogurt
1/4 cup granola
1/4 cup mixed berries (blueberries, strawberries, raspberries)

INSTRUCTIONS

1. In a serving glass or bowl, layer half of the Greek yogurt.
2. Sprinkle half of the granola over the yogurt.
3. Add half of the mixed berries.
4. Repeat the layers with the remaining yogurt, granola, and berries.
5. Serve immediately and enjoy!

Nutritional Value:
Calories: approximately 250-300 calories
Protein: 20-25 grams
Fat: 5-8 grams
Carbohydrates: 30-35 grams
Fiber: 4-6 grams

Serving Time: Breakfast or snack

Prep Time: 5 minutes

Spinach and Mushroom Frittata:
INGREDIENTS:
4 large eggs
1/4 cup milk
1 cup fresh spinach, chopped
1/2 cup mushrooms, sliced
1/4 cup diced onions
1/4 cup shredded cheese (such as Swiss or cheddar)
Salt and pepper to taste
1 teaspoon olive oil

INSTRUCTIONS:
1. Preheat the oven to 350°F (175°C).
2. In a bowl, whisk together the eggs, milk, salt, and pepper.
3. Heat olive oil in an oven-safe skillet over medium heat.
4. Add the onions and mushrooms to the skillet and sauté until softened.

5. Add the spinach to the skillet and cook until wilted.
6. Pour the egg mixture over the vegetables in the skillet.
7. Sprinkle the shredded cheese evenly on top.
8. Cook on the stovetop for 2-3 minutes or until the edges start to set.
9. Transfer the skillet to the preheated oven and bake for 12-15 minutes or until the frittata is set and lightly golden on top.
10. Remove from the oven and let it cool for a few minutes.
11. Slice into wedges and serve warm.

Nutritional Value:
Calories: approximately 150-200 calories per serving
Protein: 10-12 grams
Fat: 10-12 grams
Carbohydrates: 4-6 grams
Fiber: 1-2 grams
Serving Time: Breakfast or brunch

Prep Time: 10 minutes

Peanut Butter and Banana Smoothie:
INGREDIENTS:
1 ripe banana, frozen or fresh
1 tablespoon natural peanut butter
1 cup unsweetened almond milk (or any preferred milk)
1 tablespoon honey or maple syrup (optional)
Ice cubes (optional)

INSTRUCTIONS:
1. In a blender, combine the frozen or fresh banana, peanut butter, almond milk, and sweetener if desired.
2. Blend until smooth and creamy.
3. If desired, add ice cubes and blend again for a chilled and frosty texture.
4. Pour into a glass and enjoy!

Nutritional Value:
Calories: approximately 250-300 calories

Protein: 6-8 grams
Fat: 10-12 grams
Carbohydrates: 30-35 grams
Fiber: 4-6 grams
Serving Time: Breakfast or snack

Prep Time: 5 minutes

Veggie Breakfast Scramble:

INGREDIENTS:
2 large eggs
1/4 cup diced bell peppers (any color)
1/4 cup diced zucchini
1/4 cup diced tomatoes
2 tablespoons diced onions
Salt and pepper to taste
1 teaspoon olive oil

INSTRUCTIONS:
1. Heat olive oil in a non-stick skillet over medium heat.

2. Add the onions, bell peppers, zucchini, and tomatoes to the skillet. Sauté for 2-3 minutes until slightly softened.
3. In a bowl, whisk the eggs and season with salt and pepper.
4. Push the vegetables to one side of the skillet and pour the beaten eggs into the space.
5. Allow the eggs to cook for a few seconds until they start to set around the edges.
6. Gently scramble the eggs with a spatula, incorporating the cooked vegetables.
7. Continue cooking until the eggs are fully cooked and scrambled to your desired consistency.
8. Transfer the scramble to a plate and serve hot.

Nutritional Value:
Calories: approximately 150-200 calories
Protein: 12-14 grams
Fat: 8-10 grams
Carbohydrates: 6-8 grams
Fiber: 2-3 grams

Serving Time: Breakfast

Prep Time: 10 minutes

Avocado Toast with Poached Eggs:

INGREDIENTS:
2 slices of whole grain bread, toasted
1 ripe avocado, mashed
2 poached eggs
Salt and pepper to taste
Optional toppings: sliced tomatoes, micro greens, hot sauce

INSTRUCTIONS:

1. Spread the mashed avocado evenly on the toasted bread slices.
2. Place a poached egg on top of each avocado toast.
3. Season with salt and pepper to taste.

4. Add optional toppings like sliced tomatoes, micro greens, or a drizzle of hot sauce.
5. Serve immediately and enjoy!

Nutritional Value:
Calories: approximately 300-350 calories
Protein: 15-18 grams
Fat: 15-18 grams
Carbohydrates: 25-30 grams
Fiber: 8-10 grams
Serving Time: Breakfast or brunch

Prep Time: 15 minutes

Chapter 7: Lunch Recipes For Prostate Health

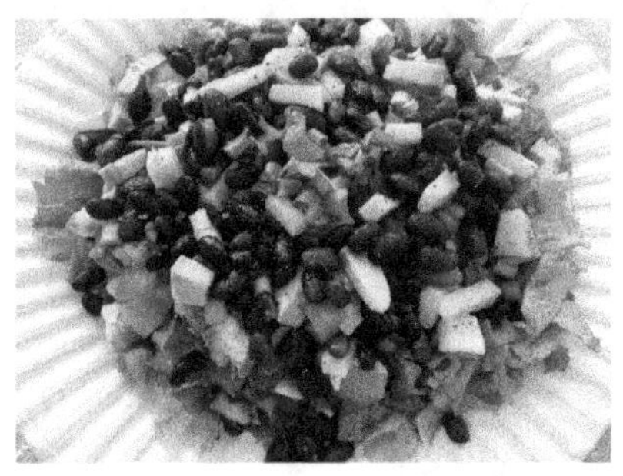

Baked Sweet Potato with Black Beans and Salsa:

Turkey and Hummus Wrap with Veggies:Grilled Vegetable Panini with Pesto:

Salmon and Quinoa Bowl with Veggies:

Greek Chicken Wrap with Tzatziki Sauce:

In this chapter, we will explore a variety of delicious and nutritious lunch recipes that are prostate cancer-friendly. These recipes are designed to incorporate wholesome ingredients that support overall health and well-being.

Baked Sweet Potato with Black Beans and Salsa:
INGREDIENTS:
1 large sweet potato
1/2 cup canned black beans, rinsed and drained
1/4 cup salsa
1 tablespoon chopped fresh cilantro (optional)

INSTRUCTIONS:
1. Preheat the oven to 400°F (200°C).
2. Wash the sweet potato and pierce it several times with a fork.
3. Place the sweet potato on a baking sheet and bake for 40-45 minutes or until tender.
4. Once cooked, split the sweet potato open and fluff the flesh with a fork.

5. Top with black beans, salsa, and chopped cilantro.
6. Serve hot and enjoy!

Nutritional Value:
Calories: approximately 300-350 calories
Protein: 10-12 grams
Fat: 1-2 grams
Carbohydrates: 60-70 grams
Fiber: 10-12 grams
Serving Time: Lunch or dinner

Prep Time: 5 minutes

Turkey and Hummus Wrap with Veggies:

INGREDIENTS:
1 whole wheat tortilla or wrap
2-3 slices of roasted turkey breast
2 tablespoons hummus
Thinly sliced cucumber
Thinly sliced tomato
Baby spinach or lettuce leaves
INSTRUCTIONS:

1. Lay the whole wheat tortilla or wrap it on a clean surface.
2. Spread the hummus evenly over the tortilla.
3. Layer the turkey slices, cucumber, tomato, and spinach or lettuce leaves on top of the hummus.
4. Roll the tortilla tightly, tucking in the sides as you go.
5. Cut the wrap in half diagonally, if desired.
6. Serve and enjoy!

Nutritional Value:

Calories: approximately 250-300 calories

Protein: 20-25 grams

Fat: 5-8 grams

Carbohydrates: 30-35 grams

Fiber: 4-6 grams

Serving Time: Lunch

Prep Time: 10 minutes

Grilled Vegetable Panini with Pesto:

INGREDIENTS:
2 slices of whole-grain bread
2 tablespoons pesto sauce
Assorted grilled vegetables (such as zucchini, eggplant, and bell peppers)
1-2 slices of mozzarella or provolone cheese (optional)

INSTRUCTIONS:
1. Preheat a panini press or grill pan.
2. Spread the pesto sauce on one side of each bread slice.
3. Layer the grilled vegetables on one slice of bread.
4. If desired, add a slice or two of mozzarella or provolone cheese on top of the vegetables.
5. Place the other bread slice on top, pesto side down.
6. Grill the sandwich in the panini press or grill pan until the bread is toasted and the cheese is melted (if using).

7. Remove from the heat and let it cool slightly.
8. Cut the panini in half or quarters, if desired.
9. Serve warm and enjoy!

Nutritional Value

Calories: approximately 300-350 calories

Protein: 10-12 grams

Fat: 10-12 grams

Carbohydrates: 40-45 grams

Fiber: 6-8 grams

Serving Time: Lunch or dinner

Prep Time: 15 minutes

Salmon and Quinoa Bowl with Veggies:

INGREDIENTS:

4-6 ounces grilled or baked salmon fillet

1/2 cup cooked quinoa

Assorted roasted or steamed vegetables (such as broccoli, carrots, and bell peppers)

Lemon wedges for garnish

INSTRUCTIONS:

1. Place the cooked quinoa in a bowl as the base.
2. Top with grilled or baked salmon fillet, flaking it into bite-sized pieces.
3. Add the roasted or steamed vegetables around the salmon.
4. Squeeze fresh lemon juice over the bowl for added flavor.
5. Serve and enjoy!

Nutritional Value:

Calories: approximately 350-400 calories

Protein: 25-30 grams

Fat: 10-12 grams

Carbohydrates: 30-35 grams

Fiber: 5-7 grams

Serving Time: Lunch or dinner

Prep Time: 15 minutes

Greek Chicken Wrap with Tzatziki Sauce:

INGREDIENTS:
1 whole wheat tortilla or wrap
4-6 ounces grilled chicken breast, sliced
2 tablespoons tzatziki sauce
Sliced cucumber
Sliced red onion
Chopped fresh parsley or dill

INSTRUCTIONS:

1. Lay the whole wheat tortilla or wrap it on a clean surface.
2. Spread the tzatziki sauce evenly over the tortilla.
3. Layer the grilled chicken slices, cucumber, and red onion on top of the sauce.
4. Sprinkle with chopped fresh parsley or dill.
5. Roll the tortilla tightly, tucking in the sides as you go.
6. Cut the wrap in half diagonally, if desired.

7. Serve and enjoy!

Nutritional Value:
Calories: approximately 300-350 calories
Protein: 25-30 grams
Fat: 6-8 grams
Carbohydrates: 30-35 grams
Fiber: 4-6 grams
Serving Time: Lunch

Prep Time: 10 minutes

Tips:

Marinate the chicken in Greek yogurt, lemon juice, and herbs before grilling for added tenderness and flavor.

Add a handful of mixed greens or baby spinach for extra freshness and nutrition.

These lunch and dinner recipes provide a balance of nutrients and flavors to support prostate health. Enjoy these delicious meals and feel nourished throughout the day!

Chapter 8: Nourishing Dinners for Comfort and Health

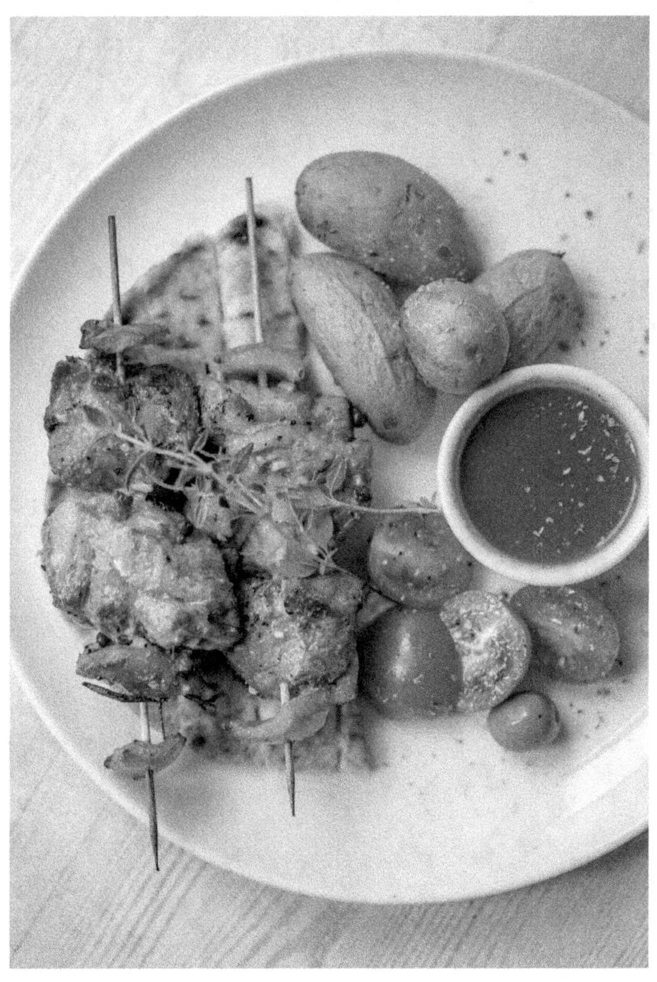

Grilled Lemon Herb Salmon

Hearty Vegetable and Bean Stew

Stir-Fried Chicken with Broccoli and Brown Rice:

Turkey Chili with Beans:

Veggie Stir-Fry with Tofu:

Grilled Lemon Herb Salmon:

INGREDIENTS:
6-8 ounces salmon fillet
1 tablespoon fresh lemon juice
1 tablespoon olive oil
1 teaspoon chopped fresh dill
1 teaspoon chopped fresh parsley
Salt and pepper to taste

INSTRUCTIONS:
1. Preheat the grill to medium-high heat.
2. In a small bowl, combine the lemon juice, olive oil, dill, parsley, salt, and pepper.
3. Brush the marinade over the salmon fillet, coating both sides.
4. Place the salmon on the preheated grill and cook for 4-6 minutes per side or until the fish flakes easily with a fork.
5. Remove from the grill and let it rest for a few minutes.
6. Serve the grilled salmon with your choice of steamed vegetables or a side salad.
7. Enjoy!

Nutritional Value:

Calories: approximately 300-350 calories
Protein: 25-30 grams
Fat: 15-18 grams
Carbohydrates: 0 grams
Fiber: 0 grams
Serving Time: Dinner

Prep Time: 15 minutes

Hearty Vegetable and Bean Stew:

INGREDIENTS:
1 tablespoon olive oil
1 medium onion, diced
2 garlic cloves, minced
2 carrots, peeled and diced
2 celery stalks, diced
1 red bell pepper, diced
1 zucchini, diced
1 can (14 oz) diced tomatoes
2 cups low-sodium vegetable broth
1 can (15 oz) kidney beans, drained and rinsed
1 teaspoon dried thyme

1 teaspoon dried oregano
Salt and pepper to taste

INSTRUCTIONS:
1. Heat the olive oil in a large pot over medium heat.
2. Add the onion and garlic, and sauté until fragrant and translucent.
3. Add the carrots, celery, bell pepper, and zucchini. Cook for about 5 minutes, stirring occasionally.
4. Stir in the diced tomatoes, vegetable broth, kidney beans, thyme, oregano, salt, and pepper.
5. Bring the stew to a boil, then reduce the heat to low and simmer for 20-25 minutes, or until the vegetables are tender.
6. Adjust the seasoning if needed.
7. Serve the vegetable and bean stew hot, garnished with fresh herbs if desired.
8. Enjoy this comforting and nutritious dinner option!

Nutritional Value:

Calories: approximately 200-250 calories
Protein: 8-10 grams
Fat: 4-6 grams
Carbohydrates: 35-40 grams
Fiber: 8-10 grams
Serving Time: Dinner

Prep Time: 15 minutes

Stir-Fried Chicken with Broccoli and Brown Rice:
INGREDIENTS:
1 boneless, skinless chicken breast, thinly sliced
2 cups broccoli florets
1 red bell pepper, thinly sliced
1 garlic clove, minced
2 tablespoons low-sodium soy sauce
1 tablespoon oyster sauce
1 teaspoon sesame oil
1 teaspoon cornstarch
Cooked brown rice for serving

INSTRUCTIONS:

1. In a small bowl, whisk together the soy sauce, oyster sauce, sesame oil, and cornstarch. Set aside.
2. Heat a tablespoon of oil in a large skillet or wok over medium-high heat.
3. Add the chicken slices and stir-fry until cooked through. Remove from the skillet and set aside.
4. In the same skillet, add a little more oil if needed, and stir-fry the broccoli, bell pepper, and garlic for 3-4 minutes until crisp-tender.
5.
6. Return the cooked chicken to the skillet and pour in the sauce mixture.
7. Stir-fry for another 2-3 minutes until the sauce thickens and coats the chicken and vegetables evenly.
8. Remove from heat.
9. Serve the stir-fried chicken with broccoli overcooked brown rice.
10. Enjoy this flavorful and wholesome dinner!

Nutritional Value:

Calories: approximately 350-400 calories

Protein: 25-30 grams

Fat: 8-10 grams

Carbohydrates: 40-45 grams

Fiber: 6-8 grams

Serving Time: Dinner

Prep Time: 20 minutes

Turkey Chili with Beans:

INGREDIENTS:

1 tablespoon olive oil

1 pound ground turkey

1 onion, diced

2 garlic cloves, minced

1 red bell pepper, diced

1 can (14 oz) diced tomatoes

1 can (15 oz) kidney beans, drained and rinsed

1 can (15 oz) black beans, drained and rinsed

1 tablespoon chili powder

1 teaspoon ground cumin

1 teaspoon paprika

Salt and pepper to taste
Optional toppings: shredded cheese, chopped
green onions, sour cream

INSTRUCTIONS:
1. Heat the olive oil in a large pot over medium heat.
2. Add the ground turkey, onion, garlic, and red bell pepper. Cook until the turkey is browned and the vegetables are softened.
3. Stir in the diced tomatoes, kidney beans, black beans, chili powder, cumin, paprika, salt, and pepper.
4. Bring the mixture to a boil, then reduce the heat to low and simmer for 30-40 minutes, allowing the flavors to meld together.
5. Adjust the seasoning if needed.
6. Serve the turkey chili hot, and top with shredded cheese, chopped green onions, or a dollop of sour cream if desired.
7. Enjoy this hearty and comforting dinner!

Nutritional Value:

Calories: approximately 300-350 calories
Protein: 25-30 grams
Fat: 8-10 grams
Carbohydrates: 30-35 grams
Fiber: 8-10 grams
Serving Time: Dinner

Prep Time: 20 minutes

Veggie Stir-Fry with Tofu:

INGREDIENTS:
1 tablespoon sesame oil
1 block (14 oz) firm tofu, cubed
2 cups mixed vegetables (such as broccoli, bell peppers, snap peas, and carrots)
2 tablespoons low-sodium soy sauce
1 tablespoon hoisin sauce
1 teaspoon cornstarch
Cooked brown rice for serving

INSTRUCTIONS:

1. Heat the sesame oil in a large skillet or wok over medium-high heat.
2. Add the cubed tofu and stir-fry until golden and slightly crisp on all sides. Remove from the skillet and set aside.
3. In the same skillet, add a little more oil if needed, and stir-fry the mixed vegetables for 3-4 minutes until crisp-tender.
4. In a small bowl, whisk together the soy sauce, hoisin sauce, and cornstarch. Pour the sauce into the skillet with the vegetables.
5. Add the cooked tofu back into the skillet and stir-fry for another 2-3 minutes until the sauce thickens and coats the tofu and vegetables evenly.
6. Remove from heat.
7. Serve the veggie stir-fry with tofu over cooked brown rice.
8. Enjoy this flavorful and protein-packed vegetarian dinner!

Nutritional Value:

Calories: approximately 300-350 calories
Protein: 15-18 grams
Fat: 10-12 grams
Carbohydrates: 40-45 grams
Fiber: 6-8 grams
Serving Time: Dinner

Prep Time: 25 minutes

These nourishing dinner recipes provide a delightful blend of flavors and nutrients to support prostate health. Whether you prefer seafood, poultry, or vegetarian options, these recipes are sure to satisfy your taste buds and nourish your body. Enjoy these comforting and healthy dinners as part of your prostate cancer-friendly meal plan!

Chapter 9: Snacks

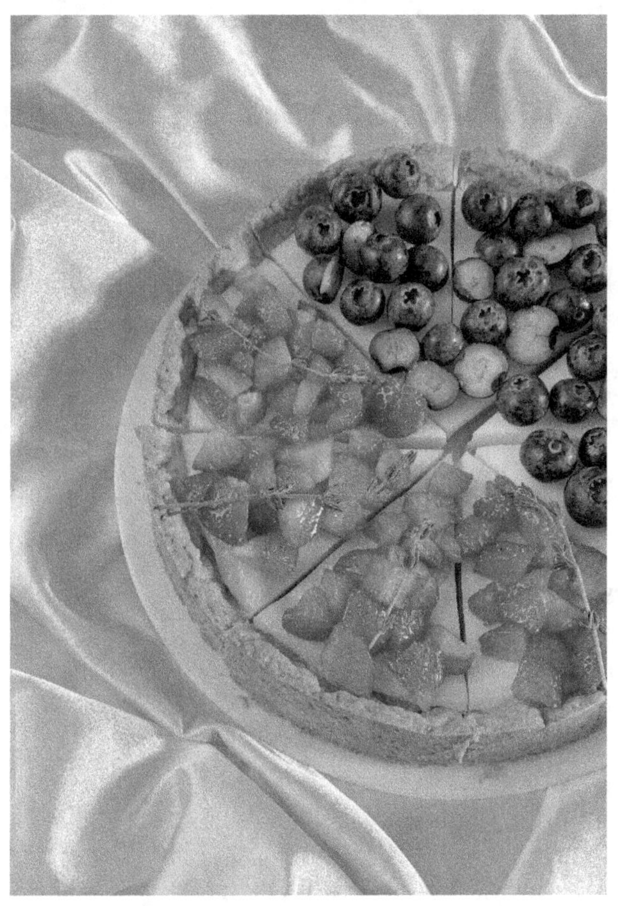

Baked Sweet Potato Fries:Air-Popped Popcorn:

Veggie Crudités with Greek Yogurt Dip:

Homemade Trail Mix:

Roasted Chickpeas with Spices:

Sometimes we crave traditional snacks that remind us of our favorite flavors and childhood memories. In this chapter, we'll explore a variety of traditional snacks that have been given a healthy twist, making them suitable for a prostate cancer-friendly diet.

These snacks are delicious, satisfying, and packed with nutrients. Let's dive in!

Baked Sweet Potato Fries:
INGREDIENTS:

2 medium sweet potatoes

1 tablespoon olive oil

1 teaspoon paprika

1/2 teaspoon garlic powder

1/2 teaspoon salt

1/4 teaspoon black pepper

INSTRUCTIONS:

1. Preheat the oven to 425°F (220°C).
2. Wash and peel the sweet potatoes. Cut them into long, thin strips resembling fries.
3. In a bowl, toss the sweet potato strips with olive oil, paprika, garlic powder, salt, and black pepper until they are well coated.
4. Arrange the sweet potato fries in a single layer on a baking sheet.
5. Bake for 20-25 minutes, flipping once halfway through, until the fries are crispy and golden brown.
6. Remove from the oven and let them cool slightly before serving.

7. Enjoy the baked sweet potato fries as a healthier alternative to traditional french fries!

Nutritional Value:

Calories: approximately 150-200 calories per 1 cup serving

Protein: 2-4 grams

Fat: 4-6 grams

Carbohydrates: 25-30 grams

Fiber: 4-6 grams

Preparation Time: 10 minutes

Air-Popped Popcorn:
INGREDIENTS:

1/2 cup popcorn kernels

Cooking spray

Salt or other seasonings to taste (such as nutritional yeast, garlic powder, or cinnamon)

INSTRUCTIONS

1. **Place the popcorn kernels in an air popper according to the manufacturer's instructions.**

2. Turn on the air popper and let it pop the kernels into light and fluffy popcorn.
3. Transfer the popcorn to a large bowl.
4. Lightly spray the popcorn with cooking spray to help the seasonings adhere.
5. Sprinkle with salt or other desired seasonings.
6. Toss the popcorn gently to distribute the seasonings evenly.
7. Enjoy the guilt-free pleasure of air-popped popcorn as a crunchy and satisfying snack!

Nutritional Value:

Calories: approximately 30-40 calories per 1 cup serving

Protein: 1 gram

Fat: 0 grams

Carbohydrates: 7-8 grams

Fiber: 1-2 grams

Preparation Time: 5 minutes

Veggie Crudités with Greek Yogurt Dip:
INGREDIENTS:

Assorted fresh vegetables (such as carrot sticks, celery sticks, cucumber slices, and cherry tomatoes)

1 cup Greek yogurt

1 tablespoon lemon juice

1/2 teaspoon dried dill

1/2 teaspoon garlic powder

Salt and pepper to taste

INSTRUCTIONS:

1. Wash and cut the vegetables into sticks, slices, or bite-sized pieces.
2. In a small bowl, combine the Greek yogurt, lemon juice, dried dill, garlic powder, salt, and pepper. Mix well to incorporate the flavors.
3. Serve the fresh vegetable crudités with the Greek yogurt dip on the side.
4. Dip the vegetables in the creamy and tangy dip for a refreshing and nutritious snack!

Nutritional Value:

Calories: approximately 80-100 calories
Protein: 8-10 grams
Fat: 0-2 grams
Carbohydrates: 10-12 grams
Fiber: 2-4 grams

Preparation Time: 10 minutes

Homemade Trail Mix:
INGREDIENTS:
1/2 cup unsalted almonds
1/2 cup unsalted cashews
1/2 cup dried cranberries
1/4 cup dark chocolate chips

INSTRUCTIONS:
1. In a bowl, combine the almonds, cashews, dried cranberries, and dark chocolate chips.
2. Mix well to ensure an even distribution of ingredients.
3. Transfer the trail mix to a resealable bag or container.

4. Carry it with you for a convenient and satisfying snack on the go!

Nutritional Value:

Calories: approximately 200-250 calories per 1/4 cup serving

Protein: 5-7 grams

Fat: 15-18 grams

Carbohydrates: 15-20 grams

Fiber: 3-4 grams

Preparation Time: 5 minutes

Roasted Chickpeas with Spices:
INGREDIENTS:

1 can (15 oz) chickpeas, drained and rinsed

1 tablespoon olive oil

1 teaspoon ground cumin

1/2 teaspoon paprika

1/2 teaspoon garlic powder

1/4 teaspoon cayenne pepper (optional)

Salt and pepper to taste

INSTRUCTIONS:

1. Preheat the oven to 400°F (200°C).

2. Pat the chickpeas dry using a clean kitchen towel or paper towel.
3. In a bowl, toss the chickpeas with olive oil, ground cumin, paprika, garlic powder, cayenne pepper (if using), salt, and pepper until well coated.
4. Spread the chickpeas in a single layer on a baking sheet.
5. Roast in the oven for 25-30 minutes, shaking the pan occasionally, until the chickpeas are crispy and golden brown.
6. Remove from the oven and let them cool slightly before serving.
7. Enjoy the savory and crunchy roasted chickpeas as a healthier alternative to traditional snacks!

Nutritional Value:

Calories: approximately 120-150 calories per 1/4 cup serving

Protein: 4-6 grams

Fat: 4-6 grams

Carbohydrates: 15-20 grams

Fiber: 4-6 grams

Preparation Time: 10 minutes

These traditional snack recipes with a healthy twist provide a balance of flavors and nutrients to satisfy your cravings. Incorporate them into your snacking routine to enjoy guilt-free indulgence while supporting your prostate health. Snack smart, stay satisfied, and enjoy these wholesome options!

Chapter 10: Indulgent Healthy Desserts

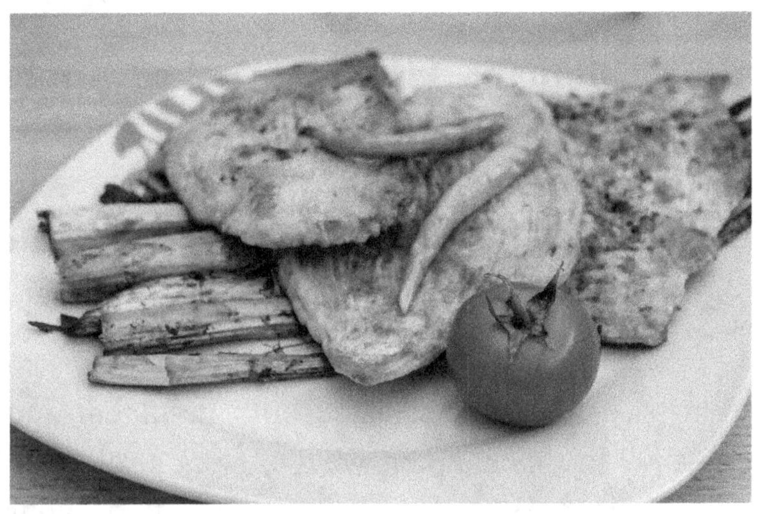

Dark Chocolate Avocado Mousse:

Berry Chia Pudding:

Frozen Banana Ice CreamBaked Apple with Cinnamon and Walnuts:

Yogurt Parfait with Fresh Berries and Almonds:

Who says desserts can't be both indulgent and healthy? In this chapter, we'll explore a selection of delicious dessert recipes that satisfy your sweet tooth while still aligning with a prostate cancer-friendly diet. These desserts are made with wholesome ingredients, and natural sweeteners, and are lower in added sugars. Let's dive into some guilt-free indulgence!

Dark Chocolate Avocado Mousse:

INGREDIENTS:

2 ripe avocados
1/4 cup unsweetened cocoa powder
1/4 cup pure maple syrup or honey
1/4 cup unsweetened almond milk
1 teaspoon vanilla extract
Pinch of salt
Optional toppings: sliced strawberries, chopped nuts, or shaved dark chocolate

INSTRUCTIONS:
1. Cut the avocados in half, remove the pits, and scoop out the flesh.
2. In a blender or food processor, combine the avocado flesh, cocoa powder, maple syrup or honey, almond milk, vanilla extract, and salt.
3. Blend until smooth and creamy, scraping down the sides as needed.
4. Transfer the mixture to serving bowls or glasses.

5. Refrigerate for at least 1 hour to allow the mousse to set.
6. Before serving, top with sliced strawberries, chopped nuts, or shaved dark chocolate if desired.
7. Indulge in this rich and velvety chocolate mousse packed with healthy fats and antioxidants!

Nutritional Value:

Calories: approximately 200-250 calories per serving

Protein: 3-4 grams

Fat: 15-18 grams

Carbohydrates: 20-25 grams

Fiber: 7-8 grams

Preparation Time: 10 minutes

Berry Chia Pudding:

INGREDIENTS:

1/4 cup chia seeds

1 cup unsweetened almond milk or coconut milk

1 tablespoon pure maple syrup or honey

1/2 teaspoon vanilla extract

Mixed berries for topping (such as strawberries, blueberries, or raspberries)

INSTRUCTIONS:
1. In a bowl, whisk together the chia seeds, almond milk or coconut milk, maple syrup or honey, and vanilla extract.
2. Let the mixture sit for 5 minutes, then whisk again to ensure the chia seeds are evenly distributed.
3. Cover the bowl and refrigerate for at least 2 hours or overnight, allowing the chia seeds to absorb the liquid and create a pudding-like consistency.
4. Before serving, give the pudding a good stir.
5. Top with a handful of mixed berries for added sweetness and antioxidants.
6. Enjoy this creamy and satisfying chia pudding as a guilt-free dessert or even a nourishing breakfast option!

Nutritional Value:

Calories: approximately 150-200 calories per serving
Protein: 4-5 grams
Fat: 7-8 grams
Carbohydrates: 20-25 grams
Fiber: 9-10 grams
Preparation Time: 5 minutes

Frozen Banana Ice Cream:

INGREDIENTS:
2 ripe bananas, sliced and frozen
2 tablespoons unsweetened almond milk or coconut milk
Optional toppings: crushed nuts, dark chocolate chips, or shredded coconut

INSTRUCTIONS:
1. Place the frozen banana slices and almond milk or coconut milk in a blender or food processor.
2. Blend until the mixture becomes creamy and smooth, resembling the texture of soft-serve ice cream. You may need to

stop and scrape down the sides as you blend.

3. Transfer the banana ice cream to a bowl.

4. Add your choice of toppings such as crushed nuts, dark chocolate chips, or shredded coconut for added flavor and texture.

5. Serve immediately and enjoy the creamy and naturally sweet frozen banana ice cream.

Nutritional Value:
Calories: approximately 100-150 calories per serving
Protein: 1-2 grams
Fat: 0-2 grams
Carbohydrates: 25-30 grams
Fiber: 3-4 grams
Preparation Time: 5 minutes

Baked Apple with Cinnamon and Walnuts:

INGREDIENTS:

1 medium apple, cored and sliced
1 teaspoon pure maple syrup or honey
1/2 teaspoon ground cinnamon
1 tablespoon chopped walnuts

INSTRUCTIONS:

1. Preheat the oven to 350°F (175°C).
2. Place the apple slices in a baking dish.
3. Drizzle the maple syrup or honey over the apple slices.
4. Sprinkle the ground cinnamon and chopped walnuts on top.
5. Bake in the oven for 15-20 minutes or until the apple slices are tender and lightly caramelized.
6. Remove from the oven and let it cool slightly before serving.

7. Enjoy the warm and comforting baked apple as a delightful dessert or even a healthy breakfast option!

Nutritional Value:

Calories: approximately 100-150 calories per serving

Protein: 1 gram

Fat: 4-5 grams

Carbohydrates: 20-25 grams

Fiber: 4-5 grams

Preparation Time: 5 minutes

Yogurt Parfait with Fresh Berries and Almonds:

INGREDIENTS:

1 cup Greek yogurt

1 tablespoon pure maple syrup or honey

1/2 teaspoon vanilla extract

Assorted fresh berries (such as strawberries, blueberries, or raspberries)

1 tablespoon sliced almonds

INSTRUCTIONS:

1. In a bowl, combine the Greek yogurt, maple syrup or honey, and vanilla extract. Mix well to incorporate the flavors.
2. In a glass or parfait dish, layer the yogurt mixture, fresh berries, and sliced almonds.
3. Repeat the layers until the glass or dish is filled.
4. Top with a few additional berries and almonds for garnish.
5. Enjoy this refreshing and protein-packed yogurt parfait as a guilt-free dessert or a healthy snack option!

Nutritional Value:

Calories: approximately 150-200 calories per serving
Protein: 15-18 grams
Fat: 4-6 grams
Carbohydrates: 20-25 grams
Fiber: 2-3 grams
Preparation Time: 5 minutes

Indulge in these healthy desserts that are packed with wholesome ingredients and natural sweetness. These recipes provide a balance of flavors and nutrients, allowing you to satisfy your sweet cravings while supporting your prostate health. Enjoy the guilt-free pleasure of these treats and embrace the goodness of a prostate cancer-friendly diet!

Chapter 11: Hydrating and Refreshing Beverages

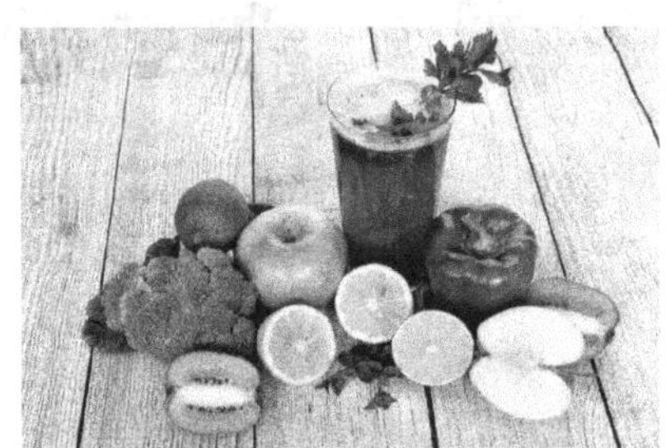

Herbal Infusion: Cooling Mint and Citrus Tea

Fruity Infused Water: Cucumber and Watermelon Splash

Nutrient-Packed Smoothie: Green Power Boost

Fresh Juice Blend: Citrus Zing

Energizing Smoothie: Berry Blast

Staying hydrated is essential for maintaining good health, especially during prostate cancer treatment. In this chapter, we'll delve into a selection of hydrating and refreshing beverage recipes that will not only quench your thirst but also provide vital nutrients to support your well-being. From herbal teas and infused waters to delicious smoothies and juices, these recipes are designed to keep you hydrated and revitalized. Let's explore the world of hydrating and refreshing beverages!

Herbal Infusion: Cooling Mint and Citrus Tea
INGREDIENTS:
2 cups water
1 tablespoon fresh mint leaves
1 lemon, sliced
1 orange, sliced
Ice cubes (optional)
Fresh mint sprigs for garnish (optional)

INSTRUCTIONS:
1. In a saucepan, bring the water to a boil.
2. Add the mint leaves, lemon slices, and orange slices to the boiling water.
3. Reduce the heat and let the mixture simmer for 5 minutes.
4. Remove the saucepan from the heat and let it cool slightly.
5. Strain the infused liquid into a pitcher or teapot.
6. Refrigerate until chilled.

7. Serve the tea over ice cubes if desired and garnish with fresh mint sprigs.

8. Enjoy the cooling and refreshing flavors of this herbal infusion!

Nutritional Value:

Calories: 0; Fat: 0g; Carbohydrates: 0g; Protein: 0g

Preparation Time: 10 minutes

Serving: Serve hot or chilled, with or without ice cubes. Garnish with fresh mint sprigs.

Fruity Infused Water: Cucumber and Watermelon Splash

INGREDIENTS:

4 cups water

1/2 cucumber, sliced

1 cup cubed watermelon

Fresh mint leaves for garnish (optional)

Ice cubes (optional)

INSTRUCTIONS:

1. In a pitcher, combine the water, cucumber slices, and cubed watermelon.

2. Stir gently to mix the ingredients.
3. Refrigerate for at least 2 hours to allow the flavors to infuse.
4. Serve the infused water chilled over ice cubes if desired.
5. Garnish with fresh mint leaves for an extra touch of freshness.
6. Sip on this hydrating and fruity-infused water to quench your thirst and revitalize your body!

Nutritional Value:

Calories: 0; Fat: 0g; Carbohydrates: 0g; Protein: 0g

Preparation Time: 5 minutes (plus 2 hours of chilling time)

Serving: Serve chilled, with or without ice cubes. Garnish with fresh mint leaves.

Nutrient-Packed Smoothie: Green Power Boost

INGREDIENTS:

1 ripe banana

1 cup fresh spinach leaves

1/2 cup sliced cucumber

1/2 cup chopped pineapple

1/2 cup coconut water

1/2 cup unsweetened almond milk

Optional: 1 tablespoon of chia seeds or flaxseeds

INSTRUCTIONS:

1. In a blender, combine the banana, spinach leaves, sliced cucumber, chopped pineapple, coconut water, and almond milk.
2. Blend until smooth and creamy.
3. If desired, add chia seeds or flaxseeds and blend for a few more seconds.
4. Pour the smoothie into a glass and serve chilled.
5. Reap the benefits of this nutrient-packed green smoothie that provides hydration and a boost of essential vitamins and minerals!

Nutritional Value:

Calories: approximately 150-200 calories; Fat: 2-3g; Carbohydrates: 30-35g; Protein: 4-5g

Preparation Time: 5 minutes

Serving: Serve chilled in a glass. Enjoy as a breakfast smoothie or a refreshing drink during the day.

Fresh Juice Blend: Citrus Zing

INGREDIENTS:
2 oranges, peeled and segmented
1 grapefruit, peeled and segmented
1 lime, juiced
1 tablespoon honey or maple syrup (optional)

INSTRUCTIONS:

1. Place the orange segments, grapefruit segments, and lime juice in a juicer or blender.
2. Process until smooth and well blended.
3. If desired, add honey or maple syrup for a touch of sweetness and blend again.
4. Pour the juice into a glass and serve immediately.
5. Experience the invigorating zing of this citrus juice blend, rich in vitamin C and natural flavors!
6. Hydrating and refreshing beverages are essential for maintaining proper hydration and supporting overall

Nutritional Value:
Calories: approximately 70-90 calories; Fat: 0g; Carbohydrates: 18-20g; Protein: 1-2g

Preparation Time: 5 minutes

Serving: Serve immediately in a glass. Enjoy as a morning pick-me-up or as a refreshing drink throughout the day.

Energizing Smoothie: Berry Blast

INGREDIENTS:
1 cup mixed berries (such as strawberries, blueberries, and raspberries)
1 ripe banana
1 cup unsweetened almond milk or coconut water
1 tablespoon honey or maple syrup (optional)
Ice cubes (optional)
INSTRUCTIONS:
1. In a blender, combine the mixed berries, ripe banana, and unsweetened almond milk or coconut water.
2. Blend until smooth and creamy.
3. If desired, add honey or maple syrup for added sweetness and blend again.
4. If desired, add ice cubes and blend for a thicker, colder smoothie.
5. Pour the smoothie into a glass and serve immediately.

6. Enjoy this energizing and antioxidant-rich smoothie as a quick breakfast option or a refreshing snack!

Nutritional Value:

Calories: approximately 150-200 calories
Fat: 2-3 grams
Carbohydrates: 30-35 grams
Protein: 3-4 grams

Preparation Time: 5 minutes

Serving: Serve chilled in a glass. Customize the sweetness and consistency by adjusting the amount of honey or maple syrup and adding ice cubes if desired. Sip on this vibrant berry blast smoothie for a burst of flavor and energy!

These beverages not only provide hydration but also offer a range of beneficial nutrients, vitamins, and antioxidants. Customize the ingredients and adjust the sweetness according to your preferences. Stay refreshed and nourished with these delightful drink options!

Chapter 12: Celebrating Special Occasions

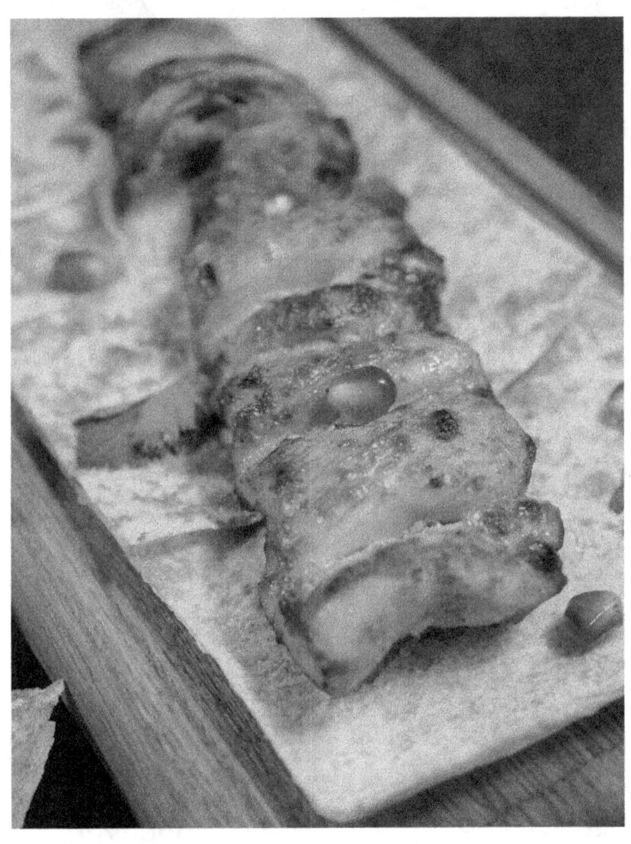

Appetizer: Smoked Salmon Canapés

Main Course: Herb-Roasted Chicken with Roasted Vegetables

Dessert: Berry and Yogurt Parfait

Beverage: Sparkling Fruit Punch

Sweet Treat: Dark Chocolate-Dipped Strawberries

Life is full of special moments that deserve to be celebrated, and prostate cancer shouldn't hinder the joy of coming together with loved ones. In this chapter, we present a collection of prostate cancer-friendly recipes that are perfect for special occasions. From festive appetizers to satisfying main courses and delectable desserts, these recipes are designed to delight the taste buds and bring people together. Let's dive into the world of celebration and create unforgettable moments!

Appetizer: Smoked Salmon Canapés

INGREDIENTS:
8 slices whole grain bread or gluten-free bread
4 ounces of smoked salmon
4 ounces of low-fat cream cheese or dairy-free cream cheese
Fresh dill for garnish (optional)
Lemon wedges for serving

INSTRUCTIONS:
1. Toast the bread slices until lightly crispy.
2. Cut each slice into smaller squares or circles to create bite-sized canapés.
3. Spread a thin layer of cream cheese on each canapé.
4. Top with a small piece of smoked salmon.
5. Garnish with fresh dill if desired.
6. Serve with lemon wedges on the side.
7. Enjoy these elegant and flavorful smoked salmon canapés!

Nutritional Value:

Calories: approximately 60-80 calories per canapé

Protein: 3-4 grams

Fat: 2-3 grams

Carbohydrates: 6-8 grams

Fiber: 1-2 grams

Preparation Time: 15 minutes

Serving: Serve the smoked salmon canapés on a decorative platter. They make a delightful appetizer for any special occasion.

Main Course: Herb-Roasted Chicken with Roasted Vegetables

INGREDIENTS:

4 bone-in, skin-on chicken breasts

2 tablespoons olive oil

1 tablespoon fresh rosemary, chopped

1 tablespoon fresh thyme, chopped

Salt and pepper to taste

4 cups mixed vegetables (such as carrots, Brussels sprouts, and potatoes), cut into bite-sized pieces
Lemon wedges for serving

INSTRUCTIONS:
1. Preheat the oven to 400°F (200°C).
2. In a small bowl, mix the olive oil, chopped rosemary, chopped thyme, salt, and pepper.
3. Place the chicken breasts on a baking sheet lined with parchment paper.
4. Rub the herb mixture evenly over the chicken.
5. In a separate bowl, toss the mixed vegetables with olive oil, salt, and pepper.
6. Arrange the vegetables around the chicken on the baking sheet.
7. Roast in the preheated oven for 35-40 minutes or until the chicken is cooked through and the vegetables are tender.
8. Remove from the oven and let it rest for a few minutes.

9. Serve the herb-roasted chicken with the roasted vegetables.
10. Squeeze fresh lemon juice over the chicken and vegetables before enjoying.

Nutritional Value:
Calories: approximately 300-350 calories per serving
Protein: 30-35 grams
Fat: 10-12 grams
Carbohydrates: 15-20 grams
Fiber: 4-5 grams

Preparation Time: 15 minutes
Cooking Time: 35-40 minutes

Serving: Plate the herb-roasted chicken with the roasted vegetables and garnish with fresh herbs if desired. Serve as a hearty main course for a celebratory meal.

Dessert: Berry and Yogurt Parfait

INGREDIENTS:

1 cup Greek yogurt
1 tablespoon pure maple syrup or honey
1/2 teaspoon vanilla extract
1 cup mixed berries (such as strawberries, blueberries, and raspberries)

1/4 cup granola or crushed nuts (optional)
Fresh mint leaves for garnish (optional)

INSTRUCTIONS:

1. In a small bowl, combine the Greek yogurt, maple syrup or honey, and vanilla extract. Mix well.
2. In serving glasses or bowls, layer the yogurt mixture with the mixed berries.
3. Repeat the layers until all the ingredients are used, ending with a layer of berries on top.
4. Sprinkle granola or crushed nuts on top for added crunch and texture, if desired.
5. Garnish with fresh mint leaves for a touch of freshness.
6. Serve immediately or refrigerate until ready to serve.

Nutritional Value:

Calories: approximately 150-200 calories per serving
Protein: 10-12 grams
Fat: 2-3 grams
Carbohydrates: 20-25 grams
Fiber: 3-4 grams
Preparation Time: 10 minutes

Serving: Serve the berry and yogurt parfait in individual glasses or bowls. It makes a light and refreshing dessert option for any special occasion.

Beverage: Sparkling Fruit Punch

INGREDIENTS:
2 cups mixed fruit juice (such as orange juice, cranberry juice, or pineapple juice)
1 cup sparkling water or Club soda
Fresh fruit slices for garnish (optional)
Ice cubes

INSTRUCTIONS:

1. In a pitcher, combine the mixed fruit juice and sparkling water.
2. Stir gently to mix the ingredients.
3. Add ice cubes to the pitcher to keep the punch chilled.
4. Pour the sparkling fruit punch into individual glasses.
5. Garnish with fresh fruit slices if desired.
6. Serve immediately and enjoy the refreshing flavors.

Nutritional Value:

Calories: approximately 80-100 calories per serving

Carbohydrates: 20-25 grams

Sugar: varies based on the fruit juice used

Preparation Time: 5 minutes

Serving: Serve the sparkling fruit punch in glasses with ice cubes and fruit garnishes. It's a festive and bubbly beverage to toast to special occasions.

Sweet Treat: Dark Chocolate-Dipped Strawberries

INGREDIENTS:
Fresh strawberries, washed and dried
Dark chocolate chips or chunks (70% cocoa or higher)
Crushed nuts or shredded coconut for coating (optional)

INSTRUCTIONS:

1. In a microwave-safe bowl, melt the dark chocolate chips or chunks in the microwave in 30-second intervals, stirring between each interval, until smooth and melted.
2. Dip each strawberry into the melted chocolate, coating about two-thirds of the berry.
3. Allow any excess chocolate to drip off, then place the dipped strawberry on a parchment-lined baking sheet.

4. If desired, roll the chocolate-dipped strawberry in crushed nuts or shredded coconut while the chocolate is still wet.
5. Repeat with the remaining strawberries.
6. Place the baking sheet in the refrigerator for about 15-20 minutes to allow the chocolate to set.
7. Once the chocolate has hardened, remove the strawberries from the refrigerator.
8. Serve the dark chocolate-dipped strawberries on a platter and enjoy!

Nutritional Value:
Calories: approximately 40-50 calories per dipped strawberry (varies based on size)
Fat: 2-3 grams
Carbohydrates: 5-7 grams
Fiber: 1-2 grams
Sugar: 3-4 grams
Preparation Time: 20 minutes (plus chilling time)

Serving: Arrange the dark chocolate-dipped strawberries on a serving platter. They make a luscious and guilt-free sweet treat for special occasions.

Celebrate special moments with these delightful and prostate cancer-friendly recipes.

Chapter 13: Exercise and Physical Activity

Particularly for older men with prostate cancer, physical exercise is essential to preserving overall health and well-being. This chapter will discuss the value of exercise and provide helpful advice and activities that are suited to the particular requirements of older men with prostate cancer. Regular physical exercise may help you build physical strength, improve your mood, and improve the quality of your life, whether you are just starting or have been active all of your life. Let's explore the world of fitness and all the advantages it may provide!

The Importance of Exercise for Seniors with Prostate Cancer:

Seniors with prostate cancer might benefit greatly from regular exercise. It helps maintain a healthy weight, maintain cardiovascular health, increase muscular strength, boost immunity, lessen tiredness, control stress, and enhance overall quality of life. Exercise may also assist with certain prostate cancer treatment side effects, such as tiredness, muscular weakness, and bone density loss. Furthermore, maintaining physical activity supports mental health and may assist seniors in keeping a good perspective during their cancer experience.

Safety Considerations:
It's crucial to speak with your healthcare provider before beginning any workout regimen. They may provide advice tailored to your unique ailment, treatment strategy, and degree of fitness. It's also crucial to pay attention to your body's signals and adjust as necessary. Start cautiously, then progressively increase the length and intensity of your exercises. To avoid injury, always warm up before the activity and cool down afterward. Stop exercising and get medical

help if required if you feel discomfort, dizziness, or shortness of breath.

Exercise Tips for Seniors with Prostate Cancer:

1. Pick workouts that you like and that are appropriate for your fitness level. Your incentive to continue the program will be increased by this.
2. To create a well-rounded fitness regimen, try to include workouts that improve your heart health, your strength, and your flexibility.
3. Include low-impact exercises like tai chi, swimming, cycling, and strolling, which are easy on the joints and have cardiovascular advantages.
4. Use resistance bands, small weights, or bodyweight movements for strength training to maintain muscle mass and strength.

5. Incorporate flexibility activities like yoga or stretching to increase joint mobility and lessen muscular tension.

6. Throughout your workouts, take pauses and relax as necessary. Do not overexert yourself; instead, pay attention to your body.

7. Before, during, and after exercise, drink water to stay hydrated.

8. Wear loose-fitting clothes and supportive shoes to promote ease of movement.

9. To boost motivation and social contact, think about working out with a buddy or signing up for a group class.

Sample Exercise Routine:

For seniors with prostate cancer, the following is an example fitness program that mixes cardio, strength training, and flexibility exercises:

a) The Warm-Up

Start by doing 5–10 minutes of mild aerobic activity, such as brisk walking or stationary cycling.
mild stretches for the main muscle groups are then performed, with each stretch being held for 15–30 seconds.

b) Exercise Your Cardiovascular System:

Select a 20–30 minute exercise you can maintain your interest in, such as cycling, swimming, or walking.
Aim for a moderate intensity where you can still talk to someone but feel a little out of breath.
c) Weightlifting:

Use small weights, resistance bands, or your body weight to do strength workouts that target the main muscle groups.
Squats, lunges, bicep curls, tricep dips, and chest presses are a few examples.

For each exercise, start with 1-2 sets of 10–12 repetitions, then over time, progressively increase the intensity and repetitions.
d) Stretching exercises:

Stretch the main muscle groups by doing stretching exercises and holding each stretch for 15–30 seconds.
Include both upper and lower body stretches, such as those for the shoulders, chest, quadriceps, and hamstrings.

e) Wind Down:

To progressively lower your heart rate, complete your workout with 5–10 minutes of low-intensity aerobic activity, such as walking or mild cycling.
additional stretches to increase flexibility and encourage relaxation are then performed.
Always pay attention to your body and modify the intensity and length of your workouts to your comfort level. Working with a certified personal trainer or another skilled fitness expert who can

provide individualized coaching and guarantee appropriate form and technique is always useful.

Conclusion: Seniors with prostate cancer may benefit greatly from regular exercise and physical activity. You may increase your general fitness, control treatment side effects, elevate your mood, and improve your quality of life by including aerobic activities, strength training, and flexibility exercises into your regimen. To guarantee your safety and well-being, always check with your healthcare team before beginning any fitness program and adjust as necessary. Enjoy the various advantages that exercise may provide by being active and optimistic.

Chapter 14: Emotional Well-being and Support

Introduction:

For seniors, dealing with prostate cancer may be emotionally difficult. Throughout your journey, it is crucial to focus on and support your mental and emotional well-being. We will look at a variety of tactics and tools in this chapter that might assist you in navigating the psychological effects of prostate cancer. There are many resources available to help your mental and emotional wellness, ranging from mindfulness exercises to support groups and therapy. Let's explore the techniques that may help you control your stress and anxiety while keeping a positive mindset.

Understanding the Emotional Impact of Prostate Cancer:

A variety of emotions, such as fear, worry, grief, anger, and uncertainty, may be triggered by prostate cancer. These feelings should be acknowledged and validated since they are a normal reaction to a serious health issue. Keep in mind that you are not alone in feeling these feelings, and asking for help may have a big impact on your well-being.

Practicing Mindfulness and Stress Management:

Exercises in mindfulness and stress-reduction methods may aid in calming the mind and reducing anxiety. Take into account the following routines:

Practice calm, deep breathing while concentrating on the feeling of the breath entering and exiting your body. By doing so, you may be able to induce relaxation in your body and lessen tension.

Meditation and visualization: Allocate a short period every day for guided meditation or visualization exercises. These techniques may help people unwind and provide a mental break from the pressure.

Yoga at chi: These mind-body exercises include relaxing motions, deep breathing, and meditation. They may aid in increasing flexibility, encouraging relaxation, and enhancing general well-being.

Hobbies and activities should be pursued: Take part in pastimes and pursuits that make you happy and aid in relaxation. This could include engaging in activities like reading, listening to music, drawing, gardening, or being outside.

Seeking Support from Family and Friends: Honest contact with your family and friends may be a great source of emotional support. Tell folks who are close to you about your thoughts, worries, and wants. Have meaningful discussions with them and let them know how they can help you out at this difficult time. An effective support network may reduce feelings of loneliness and provide a sense of warmth and understanding.

Joining Support Groups:

Consider attending a support group designed especially for men with prostate cancer. Support groups provide a secure setting where members may open up about their experiences, get support, and learn from others who have had comparable difficulties. Through local cancer organizations, hospitals, or internet resources, you may locate support groups.

Individual therapy: Seeking individual counseling may be helpful if you discover that your emotions are controlling or negatively affecting your everyday life. You may manage the psychological effects of prostate cancer with the aid of a qualified therapist or counselor who can also give coping mechanisms and assistance tailored to your requirements.

Even though experiencing a variety of emotions is natural, keeping a happy mindset may have a significant beneficial influence on your well-being. Pay attention to the parts of your life that make you happy and grateful. Take part in positive affirmation practice or positivity-promoting activities like maintaining a gratitude diary. Find supportive people and inspiring tales of prostate cancer survivors, and surround yourself with them.

In conclusion, your path with prostate cancer includes your emotional health. You may take care of your mental and emotional health by implementing techniques like mindfulness exercises, asking for help from loved ones, joining support groups, and thinking about individual therapy. Keep in mind that you are not alone in overcoming these issues and that it is OK to ask for assistance when necessary. You can handle the emotional effects of prostate cancer with resilience if you put your emotional health first and have a positive mindset.

Conclusion: Empowering Seniors on their Prostate Cancer Journey

We have gone on a gastronomic trip via this cookbook that is specially designed for seniors dealing with prostate cancer. In addition to examining the relationship between nutrition and prostate health and emphasizing the value of including superfoods, antioxidants, and phytochemicals, we have also given a broad range of scrumptious and nourishing recipes to enhance the well-being of seniors. We have spoken about the value of physical activity, mental health, and the contribution of family and friends to this journey.

It is important to underline the ability of elders to take charge of their health as we wrap out this cookbook. Seniors may improve their general health and perhaps even their quality of life by changing to a prostate cancer-friendly diet. The dishes in this cookbook not only provide seniors sustenance and taste but also give them a tool to adopt a healthy lifestyle shift.

We urge seniors to play around with the recipes, modify them to fit their dietary needs and take pleasure in the process of preparing delicious and nutritious meals. Remember to get specialized advice from your medical team, particularly if you have certain dietary limitations or medical issues.

We provide our sincere support and inspiration to all seniors starting this prostate cancer journey. Keep in mind that you are not alone. Lean on your loved ones, become involved in support groups, and go to medical experts who may provide knowledgeable counsel and aid.

Above all, embrace this path with fortitude, hope, and conviction that you can overcome obstacles. Although it may have played a role in your tale, prostate cancer does not define you. As you go down this road, embrace the strength of a good diet, regular exercise, emotional stability, and the steadfast support of the people around you.

May this cookbook be a helpful tool that nourishes, inspires, and serves as a reminder that you have the fortitude and tenacity to survive your prostate cancer journey? As you take control of your health, happiness, and tasty meals, I send my best wishes.

You can do this.

21 Day plant-based meal plan

Day 1:

> ➢ Breakfast: Overnight chia seed pudding with mixed berries and a sprinkle of chopped walnuts.
> ➢ Lunch: Quinoa salad with roasted vegetables and a lemon-tahini dressing.
> ➢ Dinner: Lentil and vegetable curry served over brown rice.
> ➢ Snack: Sliced cucumber with hummus.

Day 2:

> ➢ Breakfast: Oatmeal topped with sliced banana, almond butter, and a sprinkle of ground flaxseeds.
> ➢ Lunch: Chickpea salad sandwich with lettuce, tomato, and avocado on whole grain bread.

➤ Dinner: Roasted sweet potato and black bean tacos with salsa verde and a side of steamed broccoli.

➤ Snack: Mixed nuts and dried fruit.

Day 3:

➤ Breakfast: Vegan protein smoothie with spinach, banana, almond milk, and a scoop of plant-based protein powder.

➤ Lunch: Quinoa and black bean stuffed bell peppers with a side salad.

➤ Dinner: Whole wheat pasta with marinara sauce, roasted vegetables, and vegan meatballs.

➤ Snack: Carrot sticks with almond butter.

Day 4:

➤ Breakfast: Avocado toast topped with sliced tomato, red onion, and a sprinkle of nutritional yeast.

➤ Lunch: Lentil and vegetable soup with a side of whole-grain bread.
➤ Dinner: Vegan chili made with kidney beans, tomatoes, bell peppers, and spices, served with a side of quinoa.
➤ Snack: Apple slices with almond butter.

Day 5:

➤ Breakfast: Smoothie bowl with frozen berries, almond milk, and toppings like granola, sliced almonds, and coconut flakes.
➤ Lunch: Mediterranean quinoa salad with cucumber, cherry tomatoes, olives, and a lemon-herb dressing.
➤ Dinner: Stir-fried tofu and mixed vegetables with brown rice.
➤ Snack: Roasted chickpeas.

Day 6:

➤ Breakfast: Vegan blueberry pancakes with maple syrup and a side of fresh fruit.

- ➤ Lunch: Spinach and mushroom frittata with a side salad.
- ➤ Dinner: Vegan shepherd's pie with lentils, mixed vegetables, and mashed sweet potatoes.
- ➤ Snack: Rice cakes with almond butter and sliced strawberries.

Day 7:

- ➤ Breakfast: Acai bowl topped with granola, coconut flakes, and fresh berries.
- ➤ Lunch: Chickpea and vegetable stir-fry with brown rice.
- ➤ Dinner: Baked falafel with whole wheat pita bread, cucumber-tomato salad, and tahini sauce.
- ➤ Snack: Edamame beans.

Day 8:

- ➤ Breakfast: Quinoa breakfast bowl with mixed berries, almond milk, and a drizzle of honey.

➤ Lunch: Lentil and vegetable wrap with hummus and greens.
➤ Dinner: Roasted vegetable and chickpea quinoa bowl with a lemon-tahini dressing.
➤ Snack: Homemade trail mix with nuts, seeds, and dried fruit.

Day 9:

➤ Breakfast: Green smoothie with spinach, banana, almond milk, and a scoop of plant-based protein powder.
➤ Lunch: Vegan sushi rolls with avocado, cucumber, and carrots, served with soy sauce and pickled ginger.
➤ Dinner: Stuffed bell peppers with quinoa, black beans, corn, and salsa.
➤ Snack: Rice cakes with almond butter and sliced banana.

Day 10:

➤ Breakfast: Overnight oats with almond milk, chia seeds, and mixed berries.
➤ Lunch: Mediterranean chickpea salad with tomatoes, cucumber, olives, and a lemon-herb dressing.
➤ Dinner: Vegetable stir-fry with tofu, brown rice, and a soy-ginger sauce.
➤ Snack: Roasted beet chips.

Day 11:

➤ Breakfast: Vegan breakfast burrito with scrambled tofu, black beans, salsa, and avocado wrapped in a whole wheat tortilla.
➤ Lunch: Quinoa and lentil stuffed mushrooms with a side salad.
➤ Dinner: Spaghetti squash with marinara sauce, sautéed vegetables, and vegan meatballs.
➤ Snack: Roasted pumpkin seeds.

Day 12:

➤ Breakfast: Blueberry almond smoothie with almond milk, frozen blueberries, almond butter, and a sprinkle of flaxseeds.

➤ Lunch: Vegan Caesar salad with romaine lettuce, crispy chickpea croutons, and dairy-free Caesar dressing.

➤ Dinner: Butternut squash and lentil curry with brown rice.

➤ Snack: Fresh fruit skewers with a drizzle of dark chocolate.

Day 13:

➤ Breakfast: Vegan banana pancakes topped with sliced bananas and a dollop of coconut yogurt.

➤ Lunch: Quinoa and black bean burger with lettuce, tomato, and avocado on a whole grain bun.

➤ Dinner: Portobello mushroom steaks with roasted vegetables and a balsamic glaze.

➤ Snack: Celery sticks with almond butter.

Day 14:

➤ Breakfast: Acai smoothie bowl topped with granola, coconut flakes, and fresh berries.
➤ Lunch: Chickpea and vegetable stir-fry with brown rice.
➤ Dinner: Lentil and vegetable curry served over quinoa.
➤ Snack: mixed nuts and dried fruits 

Day 15:

➤ Breakfast: Vegan protein pancakes topped with sliced peaches and a drizzle of maple syrup.
➤ Lunch: Spinach and quinoa salad with roasted vegetables and a lemon vinaigrette.
➤ Dinner: Black bean and sweet potato enchiladas with salsa verde.
➤ Snack: Homemade kale chips.

Day 16:

➤ Breakfast: Green smoothie bowl with spinach, pineapple, coconut milk, and a sprinkle of hemp seeds.
➤ Lunch: Falafel wraps with hummus, cucumber, and tomato in a whole wheat tortilla.
➤ Dinner: Vegan chili made with kidney beans, tomatoes, corn, and spices, served with a side of quinoa.
➤ Snack: Carrot sticks with guacamole.

Day 17:

➤ Breakfast: Tofu scramble with sautéed vegetables and whole grain toast.
➤ Lunch: Lentil and vegetable soup with a side of whole-grain bread.
➤ Dinner: Veggie stir-fry with tofu, brown rice, and a teriyaki sauce.
➤ Snack: Roasted chickpeas with spices.

Day 18:

➤ Breakfast: Overnight chia pudding with almond milk, sliced almonds, and fresh berries.

➤ Lunch: Greek salad with tofu feta, tomatoes, cucumbers, olives, and a lemon-herb dressing.

➤ Dinner: Stuffed zucchini boats with quinoa, black beans, corn, and salsa.

➤ Snack: Apple slices with almond butter.

Day 19:

➤ Breakfast: Vegan breakfast sandwich with tempeh bacon, avocado, lettuce, and tomato on a whole-grain English muffin.

➤ Lunch: Quinoa and lentil salad with roasted vegetables and a balsamic vinaigrette.

➤ Dinner: Ratatouille with eggplant, zucchini, bell peppers, and tomatoes served over couscous.

➤ Snack: Trail mix with nuts, seeds, and dried fruit.

Day 20:

➢ Breakfast: Acai berry smoothie with almond milk, frozen berries, and a scoop of plant-based protein powder.
➢ Lunch: Veggie sushi bowl with avocado, cucumber, carrots, edamame, and sesame ginger dressing.
➢ Dinner: Vegan lasagna with layers of roasted vegetables, marinara sauce, and tofu ricotta.
➢ Snack: Rice cakes with almond butter and sliced strawberries.

Day 21:

➢ Breakfast: Vegan yogurt parfait with mixed berries, granola, and a drizzle of agave syrup.
➢ Lunch: Chickpea and vegetable curry served over brown rice.
➢ Dinner: Lentil and mushroom bolognese with whole wheat pasta.

➢ Snack: Roasted pumpkin seeds with sea salt.